LIVING WITH AIDS:
One Christian's Struggle
By Terry Boyd

LIVING WITH AIDS:
One Christian's Struggle
By Terry Boyd

C.S.S. Publishing Co., Inc.
Lima, Ohio

LIVING WITH AIDS: ONE CHRISTIAN'S STRUGGLE

Copyright © 1990 by
The C.S.S. Publishing Company, Inc.
Lima, Ohio

Reprinted 1992

All rights reserved. No part of this publication may be reproduced, stored in a retrieval system, or transmitted in any form or by any means, electronic, mechanical, photocopying, recording, or otherwise, without the prior permission of the publisher. Inquiries should be addressed to: The C.S.S. Publishing Company, Inc., 628 South Main Street, Lima, Ohio 45804.

9053 / ISBN 1-55673-238-4　　　　　　　　　　　　PRINTED IN U.S.A.

Dedication

I would like to dedicate this small volume to two of the most special people I have had the opportunity to know. They have allowed me to enjoy a quality of life that otherwise would have been impossible during the course of my illness. The first person is Richard. He has ridden the roller-coaster with me and has never been discouraged. He has made sure that I've taken my medication, spent countless hours with me at the hospital and seen to my every need. I would not have survived this long without his loving care.

The second is Cathie. Cathie is one of God's angels on earth. She originally encouraged me to write, and without her encouragement this book would never have been written. She has been supportive, caring, and loving — she describes it as an "embracing of souls."

I would also like to dedicate this book to the literally hundreds of people who have cared and supported me throughout. Nothing has nurtured my faith more than to know that such people exist.

And lastly, I dedicate this volume to my son and family who have shown extraordinary courage.

Table of Contents

Foreword by Cathie Lyons	9
Introduction	11
An AIDS Practicum	15
You Can't Have the Victory	
If You Don't Fight the Fight	21
I'm Going to Die!	25
Living With AIDS: A Personal Journey	31
We've Got It Wrong	37
The Joy of AIDS	41
Caring for Those Who Care for Us	45
Kurt	47
AIDS: A Manageable Disease?	49
I'm Sorry You're Dying	53
Baking Bread for the Soul	55
Earthly Attachments	57
Father	59
My Eulogy	61
Endnotes	65
For More Information	67
About the Author	69

Foreword

Terry Boyd's writings during the last year of his life represent the faith journey of a man who has no illusions. He is going to die and he knows it. The reality of death is a matter he has to deal with. In the process, Terry has developed a spirituality sufficient for the task. Herein you will read about this spiritual journey, the milestones along the way, the importance of prayer, his ability to rely on God and experience God's presence. Terry also writes about the fear, bigotry, isolation and financial hardships which too often follow a diagnosis of AIDS and which persons of faith are called to address.

"Having AIDS is just plain awful," Terry writes. "But where the Lord finds suffering in life he provides a compensating grace that somehow helps the sufferer to make it through." This compensating grace becomes for Terry the great joy of his life. Terry's book is about the miraculous power of faith in the midst of sorrow and despair, about the debilitating nature of the disease and the all-pervasiveness of God's love and grace.

Terry's belief in a life everlasting comes shining through when he writes about death, asking: "Do we really believe the promises of our religion? Do we really believe what we are told about the promises of Christ and eternal life?" Throughout his days of living with AIDS, Terry has been other-directed: concerned about the well being and feelings of loved ones and friends, concerned to let them know that his love for them will live forever and that he will see them again.

Terry confesses that he has lived with a childlike desire to really see Jesus and that he has experienced the presence of the Holy through those who have reached out to him. Terry says it best in these simple convincing words of faith: "I know Christ is present. He is there in those comforting arms. He is there in the tears. He is there in love, truly and fully. There stands my Savior." To read Terry's book is to be touched by the life of a man whose days and months of living with AIDS transformed the lives of those whose lives he touched.

Faith is a rod by which we measure a life. When I visit Terry I take a ladder. Thanks for the soul's embrace, Terry: for the "love that flows between two spirits like water in a stream." AIDS is finite. Love is infinite. AIDS has no power over the love which God has given.

                Cathie Lyons
                Associate General Secretary
                Health and Welfare Ministries Department
                General Board of Global Ministries
                The United Methodist Church

Introduction

Nearly two years ago I was told that I had AIDS. For some considerable time, I was able to continue my life as if nothing were seriously wrong. I continued to work and to lead a fairly active life. Somehow I thought that I would escape the worst of the disease and manage to squeak through. After two years, it has become fairly obvious that I'm not going to squeak through and, in fact, will face death within a relatively short time.

When I truly began to realize that I was facing death, several basic personality changes took place. First, I had to resolve this question of death; I had to tame the beast, or at least quiet it down. It has taken me this long to accomplish that task and I'm still not quite done. I would imagine that I won't be done until I actually die, but I had to find a method of finding some sort of peace. The second change was an overwhelming desire to "do something." I decided that I would attempt to write. Originally, I began to write with the idea of trying to help others who find themselves with the disease or infected by the virus. I then realized that there is much more to the story than those who have the disease. There are family members, friends, husbands, wives, children, who have to deal, somehow, with the reality that someone they love has AIDS. I quickly discovered that none of us, including professionals like ministers and counselors, are adequately prepared for coping with AIDS.

So I began my attempt to write a book. At the same time, I had been asked to write a monthly column for a church publication whose major topic was AIDS. The only conditions imposed were that the columns be two pages or less and that I try to make them as personal as possible. I continued to do research for the book, collecting quotations, reading, trying to decide what to say and how to say it. How was I going to offer something of value to someone who has found out that they are going to die? In the meantime, my collection of monthly columns expanded and became a considerable body of work. I was truly intimidated with the thought of trying to write a "real" book and was having more trouble than I had ever imagined. One morning, at 5:00 a.m., it suddenly occurred to me that I might be able to collate all of my articles into some coherent form and thereby have my book. So, I suddenly have a book, a small book. I am not a professional, so I have no means of judging its literary value or even the adequacy of its construction. I can only rely on my readers for the judgment.

During the process of collating all of the articles, I remember saying, "Gosh, this is depressing!" I guess that is because, in large portion, this is my attempt to deal with death. It sounds like I breathe and live the subject. And I did. But this was my way of coming to terms with it. I think I have been moderately successful and have recently been able to move on to other concerns. I also realized that my approach in the writing was going to present some problems to those whom I was trying to reach. Many of these articles have been written from the perspective of someone, facing death, who is also trying to justify the grand awfulness of death in terms of a Christian faith. For many persons with AIDS, religion has become such a sore point that any discussion of faith or religion is an automatic stumbling block. But I soon found that I was simply incapable of writing any other way.

Lastly, I wanted to leave something — anything. Something that might let others know who I was, what I thought, how I felt. Selfish, egotistical perhaps, but apparently not an uncommon desire for someone facing a terminal illness.

So I hope that you won't become too depressed and that my little volume may give you some insight into how one person has dealt with AIDS. And finally, I hope that it may help you to deal with AIDS in whatever form you may find it.

An AIDS Practicum

There have been a number of publications in the past several years which have attempted to offer guidance to those with AIDS on such matters as disability and insurance. I've read most of them, and for the most part they are not quite adequate. There is no substitute for experience. And in this instance, the experience can be harsh.

I was your run-of-the-mill, middle class bank employee making a reasonable salary for my area. I had a car payment, a charge account at a department store, and a VISA card that I used much too often. And then, on May 29, 1988, it was determined that I was disabled and would no longer be able to work. I had some accumulated vacation time and two weeks' salary coming. Beyond that, my income would cease. I would have no income. Of course, I knew that I should apply for Social Security Disability Benefits. Luckily, I had no difficulty in qualifying under the government's definition of "disability." The only hitch is that I did not receive any benefits immediately. And when benefits did begin, they were only about half of my previous monthly salary. No one I know could pay their normal monthly bills and expenses, plus some of the large medical costs, on a little over $700 per month.

If you feel that you may be at risk and have not yet tested positive for the virus, it is absolutely necessary that you take certain steps now. If your employer offers long-term disability insurance, make sure that you are enrolled. These plans usually insure that your disability income (with Social Security) will be a percentage of your pre-disability income, usually in the range of sixty to seventy percent. Review your medical insurance and be sure that you are acquainted with the rules of the policy regarding disability. If you have a standard policy that covers something like eighty percent, while requiring you to pay the remaining twenty percent, it may have sounded adequate when you signed up, but it just won't make it if later you become ill. My medical bills in the span of about twenty months have been well over $30,000. Twenty percent is $6,000. I don't have $6,000, but these people are going to want their money. If you can, increase your coverage or purchase a supplemental plan that will pay you in case of hospitalization, and extensive out-patient services.

In addition, there is the problem of your status with your employer if you become disabled. If you don't work, many employers consider you to have terminated. That places whatever insurance coverage you have at work in jeopardy. Originally, my medical insurance company said that they would continue to cover me for twelve months after my employment ceased. They would only cover expenses that were related to the condition that caused the disability. If I broke my leg, for example, they would not cover it. There is a federally mandated regulation called COBRA which was designed to insure that persons who had lost their jobs, for whatever reason, could continue their medical insurance for a limited amount of time — eighteen months. My insurance company emphatically stated that I was not eligible under COBRA because I was disabled. It took a high-powered attorney to convince them otherwise. So I have medical coverage for another twelve months. You will also be told that COBRA allows you to convert the policy to an individual policy before the expiration of the eighteen-month period.

I can tell you that you probably will not be able to afford the premium they will charge and that the extent of your coverage will decrease. If you retain your medical insurance under COBRA, you are responsible for the monthly premiums that your employer may have paid in whole or part while you were working. In my case, that comes to about $140 per month — another chunk out of my $700 disability payment.

Let me give you a little graphic picture:

Expenses per Month

Rent:	$198.00
Telephone:	30.00
Heat:	30.00
Electricity:	30.00
Food:	100.00
Medical Insurance:	141.50
Auto Insurance:	40.00
Car Payment:	138.50
VISA Payment:	90.00
Department Store:	40.00
Medical:	30.00 (not covered by insurance)
Total:	$868.00 Net income: $-168.00

And then there is life insurance. If you do not already have life insurance, you will not be able to get it if you test positive for AIDS or begin to have serious medical problems.

There are a number of things you can do in advance. First, on your credit accounts, or the loan of your automobile, most lenders sell credit life and disability insurance which will at least make your monthly payment should you become disabled. Buy it. It is well worth the small monthly charge. The same applies to any home mortgage you have.

Check whatever retirement plan you may have at work. Under some circumstances you may be able to withdraw a portion or the entire balance if you should become disabled. This money may be the only way that you can make it for the six months before Federal Disability payments begin.

Protect assets that you may need later just to survive. For this you need an honest family member, partner, or friend whom you can trust implicitly. Transfer your assets to this person. You should probably consult an attorney in this case because in some situations transfers of assets may disqualify you for options like Medicaid or bankruptcy. You will have to explain it in any case. Perhaps the wisest step is to pay off any debts with the money you receive from your retirement plan or the sale of assets. This won't provide you with any income, but it prevents disqualifications and reduces your monthly expenses.

Although it may seem fearful and drastic, you should also seriously consider the possibility of bankruptcy. Consider whether you will have the wherewithal and energy to handle collectors and their ilk if you become ill. It probably just isn't worth it. The bankruptcy laws were written with just this type of situation in mind, and there is no legitimate reason why you should not use them.

The question of whether to be tested is also very important for future considerations. If you have not been tested, you should not run into questions about pre-existing conditions and can feel truthful in your answers to insurance enrollment forms should you later become ill or test positive. Now this depends on your moral bent, but if you are considering being tested, make sure that you have it done anonymously and that there is no record of the results. You then have the opportunity to take some steps to protect yourself financially. While you know that you are positive, no one else will. So, if you feel comfortable with it, you can answer the insurance questions to your benefit. If there is no evidence that you knew that you were positive, the insurance company bears the burden. I'm not advocating this approach, but, when I see persons with AIDS who have no insurance, no income, sometimes even no place to live, I begin to wonder if steps such as this are really that questionable.

My last bit of advice is pretty standard, but vitally important. You should appoint an Attorney-in-Fact (through a *durable* power of attorney); you should also have a durable power of attorney for health care, papers appointing a guardian, and a will. The durable power of attorney allows whomever you appoint to take care of your bank account and monthly bills. The durable power of attorney for health care allows the person you appoint to make medical decisions for you should you be unable to do so. A guardianship allows your guardian to provide for your support and care should you be unable to do this yourself. State law varies regarding these matters, but in most states a reputable attorney can take care of these matters for a very small fee. There is a compelling reason for these documents when considering AIDS. It was not too long ago that many persons with AIDS woke up one morning with a temperature, went to the hospital, were diagnosed with pneumocystis pneumonia, and were dead within days or weeks. That is no longer the case. With the improvement in treatment, you could very well end up in the hospital for months on end, attached to every medical device imaginable. For some of us, that prospect is worse than the disease itself. And, it will most likely happen if you don't make provisions in advance.

    These are not pleasant decisions, and you may wish to avoid them. But you should know that, if you do avoid them, you do so at your own peril. AIDS is a messy, smelly, painful affair. We need to do whatever we can to reduce the suffering whenever possible. That includes financial suffering. And the major responsibility is ours, those of us who have the disease or who are at risk.

You Can't Have the Victory If You Don't Fight the Fight

For some long months, I approached my relationship with my church and others from a defensive stance. I had AIDS, and now I was at the mercy of others. Would they be accepting, compassionate, or even just polite? I worried, needlessly it appears, about rejection by those who would turn away out of fear or moral judgment. And then there were those in the church, including ministers, who would suddenly become patronizing. "Oh, you poor dear!" You know the kind of person I mean. They will tell you how sorry they are and, just as suddenly (within a fraction of a second), be talking to someone else about Mrs. Jones' pregnant daughter with their backs turned toward us. They've completed their obligation and can move on to subjects with which they are much more comfortable. The irony is that they wouldn't even have made that slight gesture if they hadn't been in church.

I took what I could get, however. Sometimes, even an insincere gesture seemed better than none at all.

Well, I've changed my tune considerably. I've already fought this disease much too long to meekly accept all that is wrong with society's (and the church's) response to AIDS. I'm afraid I've become a little abrasive — and I don't feel guilty about it. For those who are prone to judgment and who may feel that AIDS is some sort of retribution: "people who live in glass houses. . . ." Frankly, whatever sins I may have committed are none of their business. I don't barge into their spiritual/moral lives, and they should stay out of mine. My sins and transgressions are between me and my God. Of course, the church feels a little differently.

You know, I would be more willing to accept the guidance of the church in these matters if their houses were in order, and if they didn't make mistakes just like the rest of us. But we all know that they have made some tremendous blunders. Take, for example, the Roman Catholic Church, which recently convened a conference on AIDS at the Vatican. According to them, the use of preventative sexual techniques promotes promiscuity and increases the incidence of AIDS. Sorry folks, but that is one of the silliest things I've ever heard. And on top of that, no Catholic whom I know, who has been affected by AIDS, will pay any attention. Reeds in the wind.

I do not mean to say that the church has nothing to offer; it does. But, unfortunately, they have been too slow. The six-month process of dealing with the Social Security Administration has been no worse than dealing with my local conference. It is often a matter of "hurry up and wait." Well, I'm getting tired of it, especially since I don't have much time left. So I have become abrupt, impatient, sometimes obnoxious. I write letters to the editor, I go to meetings and ask why this or that hasn't been done, I write letters to the bishop, I generally cause trouble. I'm not particularly popular.

Elizabeth Taylor recently made a telling statement which was published in our local newspaper. She said that it was a shame that often the only way people come to join the battle is when they lose someone to AIDS — my experience exactly. And, I don't reserve my criticism for people who don't have the disease. Those of us with AIDS have a tremendous responsibility. This is not the time of life to retreat and to become silent. There are no more effective advocates than those who actually have AIDS. We have the responsibility to speak out, stand up, and fight. We have to become terrible boors and talk about AIDS, even when those around us don't want to hear about it. You should be prepared, however, for a decline in invitations to cocktail parties.

I had a very meaningful experience recently. I have always been a fan of Peter, Paul and Mary. For my birthday I got to see them in concert. Just before the concert, I had gone to the restroom. As I hobbled back down the aisle with my cane, the concert had already begun. The first song: "No Easy Walk to Freedom." Later, one of their songs contained the line, "You can't have the victory if you don't fight the fight."

I'm Going to Die!

I remember quite well that paralyzing fear I experienced when the doctor told me that I had tested positive for the human immune deficiency virus (HIV). It was really more than fear; it was sheer panic. I was totally immobilized. Everything else was blotted out, and I could only see the great, dark, terrible certainty that I was going to die. I could think of nothing else; it occupied my every waking thought. My mind was a phonograph record caught in one groove, playing the same few bars over and over.

I cried, I moaned, I complained, I grieved. Whatever faith I thought I had, suddenly disappeared, and I was not favorably disposed to conversations about the Christian hope of eternal life. I was dealing with something that was slightly more concrete than a preacher's theological "pie in the sky." It was not a pleasant experience to be around me.

But life is a process of discovery, and I was still living. Slowly it began to dawn on me that I was not going to die "right now." Each morning, I would wake up and the sun would come up, and I began to realize that it was a little premature to be picking out caskets.

I still think about dying, almost every day. But death and I have reached an uneasy truce. Right now, I don't bother it, if it doesn't bother me. There is no easy way to get through this period and reach this uneasy truce with death. There are no platitudes or sugarcoated pills that will make it easy or palatable. It was just one of those things that I had to do, on my own, like the times when I was a child and I had been caught in a lie and there was no possible way of squirming out of it. I knew that I had to face the music and that there was no one who could help me.

I soon found out that there are stages of HIV disease and that there were a lot of labels. There was ARC, and full-blown AIDS, and being seriopositive. There were PWA's (Persons with AIDS) and PLA's (Persons Living with AIDS). Besides being irritating, these labels don't count for much in my book. Dealing with death seems to apply to all, whether you are seriopositive, or you have ARC, or you have full-blown AIDS, or you are a person with or a person living with AIDS.

My own experience taught me that this phase does pass. I began to realize that whatever personal or religious significance I had attached to my own death did not matter so much as the significance I attached to *living* what time remained.

In his book, *AIDS, the Spiritual Dilemma*, John E. Fortunato describes learning that he had the Epstein-Barr virus, and describes one of his conversations with his doctor:

> "So I'm not dying!" I said to him. "Death?" [Dr.] Schlicter said disdainfully. "The hell with death. You only have two choices: living or not living. Take your pick."[1]

The question of death presented some serious roadblocks to successfully coping with the diagnosis of AIDS. Yes, it is tragic — yes, it is terrible — yes, it is sad. But that is not the entire cake; it is only one slice. I have spoken to a number of church groups about AIDS, and in some ways the initial meeting is humorous and slightly sad. They are thinking that this young man standing before them has a fatal disease. Many cannot help but sit, with their mouths hanging open, in astonishment that I am standing in front of them and that I have a smile on my face. They are thinking about death. My job, then, is to bring them to a realization of what it is like to *live* with AIDS. Death, however, is a hand tool — it gets people's attention very effectively. And you need to get their attention if they are to understand the real issues involved. Death becomes a problem when we can't move beyond it, when we ignore the needs of living persons. There are so many more important considerations. How will I love my life? In despair, in hope, in service, in fear? How will I be judged when death does come?

Again, quoting Fortunato:

> *Against the confusing spiritual backdrop of the United States in the 1980s . . . AIDS made its entrance. Most everyone would agree that it could not have come at a worse time. Here we had almost succeeded in obliterating death from our consciousnesses. We had worked so hard and for so long. More than a century of progressively hiding the Grim Reaper, of euphemizing death, of phoneying up corpses, of putting fake grass around the hole and leaving before the box was lowered. We had almost secreted ourselves from death, almost antisepticized it. And we were within a hair's breadth of our goal.*[2]

I don't want to put fake grass around my death and leave before the box is lowered. It is a fact of life. I just didn't think that I would have to come to terms with death quite so soon. During the first few months after my diagnosis, I discovered that there are "wolves in the forest," people who told me that I should not think about death at all. Such reflection is not a "positive" thing to do, and negative thoughts would only further harm my health. I don't see how anyone affected by this disease could possibly avoid thinking about death. Not only is it unavoidable, but it is necessary in order to reach some sort of peace with the idea. If I didn't, it would become so much unfinished business, always underfoot, haunting my every move.

> *I do not mean to make light of death. Whether life is good or bad, death is so awesome and terrifying that the sooner we use our faith to come to terms with it, the better off we are. But finally, death is more friend than foe.*[3]

• • •

> *I will make a stab at a "nonrational" answer to the why of AIDS. And it is this. If our journey with AIDS serves to bring us all home to the grand and grave, the joyful and sobering truth of our mortality; if this suffering helps heal the madness of an eternally empty later whose existence we have duped ourselves into believing in; if this nightmare brings back to our consciousness the resurrection hope without which life is just so much courageous despair, then in this groaning of creation, with tears and sighs, perhaps the Holy Spirit will usher in some modicum of peace or even a corner of salvation that might otherwise have been unattainable. And in that travail, perhaps . . . perhaps we will glimpse the meaning of AIDS for our spiritual journeys.*[4]

There are other fears besides the fear of death, like demons — poking, prodding, never allowing much peace. I recall my initial fear that "someone would find out," specifically my employer. For me, this fear did not appear after my fears of death. It began at the same time, and it seemed infinitely worse to live with the disapproval and judgment of those I worked with than to die. I thought to myself that it would be much easier if I just died then. At least I wouldn't have to face my boss. I even had fantasies about how I would die. Maybe I would get lung cancer. Lung cancer, or any cancer, seemed much more attractive than AIDS. I would have rather had cancer or even been run over by a bus — and of course, there was always suicide.

I could hear the thoughts of others. "Only two types of people get AIDS: homosexuals and drug users." So not only did I have AIDS, but I was afraid that others would simply assume that I was either a homosexual or that I used drugs. Neither possibility seemed to generate much feeling of security about my job.

I had more trouble with the fear of disclosure than I ever had with the fear of death. But I found out that there is only one way to deal with it. I disclosed, to everyone, to my pastor, my friends, my family, anyone who mattered to me. I found out that not everyone was going to judge or turn and run away screaming. These are the folks who have helped me to live. These are the angels of God who have helped me to overcome my other fears. These are the people who have sat patiently with me while I have cried. I could not do without them — they have become as important as food.

To me this is the essence of the Gospel imperative to "Love one another." The faith that I thought I had lost when I was diagnosed has returned. It is a gift that has been returned to me in greater measure than I ever could have imagined. To see God, you need look no further than your pastor, or your boss, or your friends who have all said that they will do whatever they can to help.

All of my little fears and worries are a lot like pesky little goblins that I have to pen up, each in its own little cage. I've taped a note to each cage with my thoughts and feelings and how to deal with each one. But then I would reach some milestone, like beginning to take the drug AZT. I had to take a toxic drug every four hours around the clock. The goblins would begin to squeak and rattle their cage doors, especially at the 2:00 a.m. dose.

Soon the drug began to affect my blood counts, and my dosage was cut in half. I had unconsciously come to think of the drug as the only thing keeping me alive. So, when my dosage was cut in half, the goblins actually broke out of their cages and it was a few days before I had them all corralled once again.

I've had to add more cages since then — the goblins multiply, you know. There was the milestone of quitting work and becoming officially disabled. How will I pay the bills, how will I live on my small disability payment, what will I do with my time besides chasing goblins?

I was a little overwhelmed. But I could only deal with one goblin at a time. I began to realize, as Fortunato says,

"In order to hear God you first have to shut up." And in order to achieve some sort of peace, I had to rely on my God.

> When we've placed our burden on the only shoulders that can take it, we'll discover that it's light and bearable and that we have what we need to carry it.[5]

The Lord, after all, is the ultimate goblin tamer.

Living With AIDS: A Personal Journey

I vividly recall a night in December or January about a year ago. It was 6:00 p.m., very cold, and getting dark. I was waiting for a bus to take me home, and I was standing behind a tree for protection from the wind.

I had recently lost a friend to AIDS. From whatever measure of intuition God had given me, I knew suddenly and quite certainly that I also had AIDS. I stood behind the tree and cried. I was afraid. I was alone and I thought I had lost everything that was ever dear to me. In that place, it was very easy to imagine losing my home, my family, my friends, and my job. The possibility of dying under that tree, in the cold, utterly cut off from any human love seemed very real. I prayed through my tears. Over and over, I prayed: "let this cup pass." But I knew. Several months later, in April, a doctor told me what I had discovered for myself. Now it has been nearly a year. I am still here, still working, still living. I go to the doctor once a month and find myself reassuring him that I feel quite well. He mutters to himself and rereads the latest laboratory results which show my immune system declining toward zero.

When I was growing up, I literally detested grubby, down-in-the-dirt sorts of work like cleaning the garage or working in the garden. Later, a friend who was a psychiatrist suggested that I accept a summer job at a lumber camp in the Northwest. He chuckled with glee and suggested it might be a constructive emotional experience. I escaped that one. This last year, though, has been a constructive emotional experience. Parts of it have been grubby and down-in-the-dirt, and other parts have been life changing. I cry more now. I laugh more now, too.

I have come to realize that my story is not in any way unique, nor is the fact that I will most likely die within two or three years. Like many of my brothers and sisters, I have had to come to terms with my own death, and the deaths of many of those I love.

My death will not be extraordinary. It occurs daily to others just like me. And I have realized that death is not really the issue at all. The challenge of having AIDS is not dying of AIDS, but living with AIDS. I didn't come to these realizations easily and, unfortunately, wasted precious time caught up in what I thought was the tragedy of my impending demise.

I still have a difficult time when someone I love is sick, in the hospital, or dies. We have all been to far too many funerals, and many of us don't know how we will be able to find any more tears for the friends we continue to lose. In a story published recently about a man who lost a close friend to AIDS, the author says that after his friend died, he thought that just maybe the horror was over; that somehow it would all go away and everything could get back to the way it once was. But, just as he starts to think the horror is over, the telephone rings. I am holding back tears as I write this because I have a very vivid picture of my family making those same telephone calls.

One of the major myths of the AIDS crisis is that all we need is more money to throw at the problem. Money, by itself, will not solve the problems of suffering, isolation and fear. You do not need to write a check: you need to care. If you do care, the check will follow naturally enough. But first, you have to care.

You may ask, "What can I do?" The answer is simple. You can share a meal, you can hold a hand, you can let someone cry on your shoulder, you can listen, you can just sit quietly with someone and watch television. You can hug, and care, and touch and love — even though you may be frightened of the disease.

Several years ago, I had a friend whose name was Don. I knew that he had been seriously ill. It seemed like he was in and out of the hospital with a strange assortment of ills and that he just wasn't getting any better. Finally, the doctors diagnosed AIDS. By the time he died, he had dementia and was blind. When his friends found out that he had AIDS, many did not visit him in the hospital. Yes, that included me. I was afraid — not of catching AIDS — but of death. I knew that I could be looking at my own future. I thought I could deny it, ignore it, and it would go away. It didn't. The next time I saw Don was at his funeral. I am ashamed, and I know that none of us are exempt from the sins of denial and fear. If I had a wish, it would be that no one would have to experience the death of a loved one before they realize the extent and seriousness of AIDS. What a terrible, terrible price to pay.

"What happens," you may ask, "when I get involved and I come to care about someone, and then they die?" The answer is not easy. But you may understand the importance of becoming involved, as a Christian, as a human being, regardless of the pain that may result. I have a friend whose brother recently died of AIDS. She once told me that she was always amazed to see me and to see how well I was doing. She said that she was convinced that I continued to do so well because of the love and support I have received from those around me. She then said that she knew that her brother would have lived much longer if he had received the same care and support, and if he had not felt so alone and isolated. I know that the love and care that I have received has literally kept me alive.

How many people do you know who have saved a life? I tell you that I know quite a few. You may ask, "What did they do, save a child from a burning building?" No, not exactly. "Well, did they pull someone out of a river?" Not Quite. "Well, what did they do?" When so many others are so afraid, they will sit next to me, they will shake my hand, they will hug me. They tell me that they will do all that they can to make things easier for me. Knowing people, Christians, like this has made my life a daily miracle. You can save a life, too. That life may only last for a few months, or a couple of years, but you can save it just as surely as if you had pulled someone out of the river's current.

In my earlier days, when I first "got religion," there were a few topics which fascinated me: mainly those which dealt with the presence of Christ in the modern world. We believe, for example, that Christ is present at the Eucharist. And in the service of Communion, a very short statement, but perhaps the most important, is when the minister presents us with Communion saying, "The Body of Christ." I was also quite taken with certain passages in Matthew where someone asks Jesus, "When, Lord, did we ever see you hungry and feed you, or thirsty and give you a drink? When did we ever see you a stranger and welcome you in our homes?" Jesus replies, "I tell you, whenever you did this for one of the least of these, you did it for me." And again, in Matthew, the statement that: "for where two or three come together in my name, I am there with them." I was, and probably still am, a religious innocent. I still harbor a childlike desire to really see Jesus, talk with him, ask him a few questions. So the question of when and where Christ is truly present has always been important to me.

I can tell you truthfully that I have seen Christ. When I see someone holding a person with AIDS who is crying desperately, I know I am in the presence of holiness. I know Christ is present. He is there in those comforting arms. He is there in the tears. He is there in love, truly and fully. There stands my Savior.

But finally, you will be called upon to grieve; yet, you will know that you have made a difference, and you will realize that you have gained more than you could ever have given. An old, old story really . . . about 2,000 years old.

There is a song, whose words say in part:

> *Ashes to ashes,*
> *dust into dust.*
> *Buildings will crumble*
> *bridges will rust.*
> *Mountains will disappear,*
> *rivers will dry up.*
> *So it goes with everything but love.*

Most Christian writers who have addressed the issues surrounding AIDS agree that AIDS represents a true challenge to our commitment to the concepts of love and compassion as taught by Christ. How do we respond with love and compassion in the face of such fear?

I never would have imagined that I would be truly in need of the compassion and care of my church. Not just in a philosophical sense, but in a very real sense. Church, after all, was Communion, maybe an occasional bingo game or fish fry, sometimes a youth baseball game. I had not realized the importance of the church in my life until I thought I was in danger of losing it. It was very easy to imagine the church turning away from me in fear. I imagined that no one would sit next to me on Sunday, that there would be objections to my sharing the Communion Cup, that my pastor would become cold and distant. I was terrified. It seemed that I had already lost so much, and now I would lose the church.

I was not prepared for the reality. How many of us truly believe that Christ is present in his church? How many of us recognize grace when it appears? How many of us are prepared for the love of God when it is shown to us?

Everyone in my church knows that I have AIDS. During the Passing of the Peace, I get bear hugs — not just polite handshakes. I cannot count the number of cards and telephone calls and offers of help. My pastor calls at least once a month. I think I have even become a source of pride to the congregation. They have met the monster AIDS and have decided that they are not afraid. They care about me, and they are justly proud of their ability to show love and compassion in the face of this terrible disease. And I am proud of them. AIDS has brought the congregation together and made real the ideas we have heard in so many sermons on so many Sundays.

One final story. Soon after I discovered that I had AIDS, a member of my family brought home a small packet of seeds. They were sunflowers. We lived in an apartment with a small patio with a bare patch of earth — really more of a flower box than any sort of garden. He said that he was going to plant the sunflowers in the "garden." Okay, I thought. Our luck with growing things had never been tremendous, especially with such large plants in such a small plot of ground. And I had much more important fish to fry. I was, after all, dying of AIDS, and I have never paid much attention to anything as mundane as flowers in a flower box.

But the seeds were planted and they took hold. By summertime, they stood at least seven feet high with glorious, bright yellow blooms. The blossoms followed the sun religiously, and the patio became a hive of activity as bees of all descriptions hovered relentlessly around the sunflowers. Out of row upon row of apartments which were indistinguishable from one another, it was always easy for me to spot our patio with those great halos of yellow towering high above the fence. How precious those sunflowers became. I knew I was coming home: home to those who loved me. When I saw those sunflowers, I knew that everything, in the end, would be all right.

For those of you who can find the courage to show love and compassion to someone with AIDS, I would like it very much if you could come to my house. We wouldn't do a whole lot. We would just sit on kitchen chairs, have some iced tea, and watch the bees in the sunflowers.

We've Got It Wrong

It is discomforting to realize that, after about twenty years, you have got it all wrong. Particularly in my situation, when I know that I will die before my normal time, and when I have seen so many of my friends die before me.

I've heard the phrase so many times, I'm starting to get sick of it: We all are going to die. Yeah, but no one really believes that. Death is simply not what we believe it to be; not only have I got it wrong, but so has everyone else.

I've made two resolutions recently: First, I'm done with mourning. It takes too much energy, and if I haven't understood it yet, I never will. Frankly, I have better things to do than worry about death. Second, I'm done with thinking what a terrible tragedy death is. That's part of where I had it wrong.

Death is not terrible, death is not tragic, death is not extraordinary. Death is a prime example of Christians talking out of both sides of their mouths. Do we really believe the promises of our religion? Do we really believe what we are told about the promises of Christ and eternal life? We say we do, but our words are unconvincing. Well, I've decided that I do, probably because I don't have any better choice. So all of this agonizing about death has become a monumental waste of time.

The real problem with death is those who are left behind, those who love us, those who cannot imagine life without us, husbands, wives, children, friends, lifetime partners to whom we have become a part of the very fabric of life. In that position, we cannot imagine how we will be able to bear the loss or how we will be able to continue without our beloved. We realize that the loss will cause drastic changes, and we are not sure that we are able to handle the changes. This is the problem of death, not our own individual passing to a world which we have been promised by our Savior. In effect, the problem is connected to the basic tenets of our religion. Are we to be self-directed or other-directed? Are we going to worry about ourselves or our neighbors? Our normal method of approaching our own deaths is perhaps one of the most selfish exercises I've ever seen. And I've done it myself.

It is high time that those of us who are facing death face up to our convictions and try to make some provisions to ease the loss that will come after. We have to insure that those who love us understand our feelings about death, that we do not consider it an unalterable end and that we will see them again. We have to make sure that they understand that we love them, and that nothing (not even death) can take that love away from them. We must assure them that we will be with them in spirit for as long as they remain on earth, and that they will never be alone. We must convince them that Christ was not just talking through his hat, and that it is time for them to take him into their hearts and believe, really believe. And then, somehow, we must convince them to rejoice with us and to give thanks.

I know, that last may seem to be asking quite a lot. But let me tell you how the Lord works. I've faced some pretty debilitating and unpleasant side effects of this disease called AIDS. But there has never been a new, painful development that hasn't followed with some sort of joyful blessing. Prayers of thanksgiving and praise are the only ones I know how to say anymore. And those who are left behind and who are grieving must understand this. Out of their grief and loss can come peace and joy if only they open themselves to it. Imagine yourself at a funeral and praying, Glory Be to God in the Highest! The idea may seem foreign to you, but it isn't to me. I've prayed the same prayer in the midst of a biopsy for cancer. How could I do that? Because there were no less than twenty or thirty people praying for me at that very moment. Because I had so many get well cards, I hadn't had time to open them all. Because the telephone in my hospital room never stopped ringing. Because I was never alone. I was blessed and I knew it.

If you are facing a life-threatening or terminal illness, you may think that this is not a time when you need any more responsibility. Wrong — you have more now than ever before. Your primary responsibility is to those around you, those you love. I think that we should realize that we are big boys and girls now and take the Christian responsibility that salvation imposes.

The Joy of AIDS

I suppose that some folks may be surprised, some even shocked, by the title, "The Joy of AIDS." They may wonder what kinds of joy can be associated with having a fatal and often debilitating disease. Others may wonder how there can be joy in having AIDS when they consider the fear, bigotry, financial hardship, and isolation that can result from a diagnosis of AIDS.

I would say to these folks, let's understand one another. Having AIDS is not a rock-and-roll time. It is painful (both physically and emotionally), dirty, smelly, and just plain awful. But, like so much else in life, where the Lord finds suffering he provides a compensating grace that somehow helps the sufferer to make it through. In my case, this compensating grace has been the great joy of my life. In addition, the power of the Lord to be present in an individual's life, and to really make good on all of his promises, didn't really mean a lot to me until I learned that I had AIDS. What I mean to say is that I don't think I really believed all of those Sunday sermons. A spiritual power from heaven that will give you the strength to face suffering and death? No, I didn't really believe it. It was just something that preachers were supposed to talk about, and I only saw the preacher once a week anyhow.

So, how do I know that God has intervened in my life? Easy. The first time I was in the hospital, a nurse came into my room, looked me right in the eye, and said, "How *are* you, hon?" No one could miss the care and concern in those eyes. Not what I expected. I expected that no one would want to come into my room. I had heard the stories about dinner trays being left on the floor in the hallway. And this nurse was not the exception; her attitude and sincerity were the rule.

And then there was church. I expected a whole lot of trouble there. I could see myself sitting on a pew with at least two bodies' length between me and anyone else. I pictured objections to my sharing the Communion cup. It has happened before; I've read about it. So imagine my reaction when at the Passing of the Peace, people I had known only slightly wanted to give me a hug. And then there were the countless greeting cards, telephone calls, letters. I thought, if this keeps up I'll need a secretary.

Most persons living with AIDS eventually have to deal with their "retirement" from work. Along with the financial hardship involved, there is the question, "What am I going to do — hour after hour — each day? Sit on my behind and watch television, or just wait for death?" No — here comes the Lord. First, I asked to serve on my Conference's AIDS Task Force, and then I met Cathie Lyons, the Associate General Secretary of the Health and Welfare Ministries Department of the United Methodist Church, who is responsible for producing a monthly publication on AIDS issues. And now I'm writing a monthly column. Me, a columnist? Who would have thought? Then I was asked to serve on the board of directors of an organization that provides low-cost housing to persons with AIDS. I was appointed to the finance committee and appointed co-director of volunteers. I have been asked to speak to church groups, Methodists, Presbyterians, Catholics. And somewhere I found the "push" to start writing for other publications, and to even consider this book. The book is finally done, and I have had several articles published. Writing was something that I had wanted to do since I was a teenager, but I never thought that anyone would actually want to read what I had written.

I was one of those odd products of the sixties: slightly rebellious, always bull-headed. People were not exactly my thing. I'd rather be reading or listening to the Beatles than dealing with another "person." Coming to AIDS with a disposition like that made me a prime candidate for the isolation I mentioned earlier. But, again, here comes the Lord. How can you refuse a hand extended to you in love and concern? I found that I couldn't. I now have many friends, good friends. Joy.

I've changed. And to be honest, I'm not sure that I really wanted to change. But it seems that I didn't have much choice. The Lord said, "You'll do this and I will send you this human angel to help you do it!" Joy!

A holdover from my teenage years was my relationship with my parents. My mother and father were divorced when I was about fourteen. My father just disappeared and the war was on with my mother. At one point, I had not seen or talked with my father for fifteen years. Of course, none of us had ever said, "I love you." My father just called, again, to wish me a happy birthday, and he said "I love you." My mother calls weekly, and we have found it very easy to say "I love you." See the Lord at work.

I wish that I didn't have AIDS. But, to be honest, I couldn't imagine life without the blessings God has given me, all somehow connected with having AIDS. There is joy in suffering, especially if you are a believer.

Caring for Those Who Care for Us

I have a very special friend: a "buddy." He has done my laundry and sat with me all day in the emergency room after working a midnight shift. He has cleaned, cooked, and cried with me. There are many times when I thought I could not have survived without his loving care.

During one particularly difficult period when I was extremely weak, dehydrated and losing weight at an alarming rate, he would attempt to get me to eat — something, anything. I was wasting away: a reality experienced by many persons living with AIDS.

I began to view his constant pleas for me to eat as nagging. Resentful of being treated like a child, I would remind him that I was an adult, able to make decisions for myself, and that he simply did not understand the nausea I was feeling. We went through this routine countless times. Finally, I said I would not tolerate it any more and I asked him to keep his opinions to himself. My anger and frustration were met with the same response from him.

Then, it finally began to sink in. I had never considered the anger, frustration, and real pain that someone in his position of care-provider must experience. Not only was he caring for me during a very rough period, he had lost other friends to AIDS and had seen his sister die from cancer.

I was shocked to realize how self-centered I had become. It is easy for someone with AIDS to be lulled into thinking that he or she is the center of all things. In my case, I have a very well organized support system: people from church, family and friends. At some point, I started to believe that the world revolved around me and my disease. It is a dangerous trap. My anger at my friend's attentiveness has only increased his pain, his frustration, his anger. I realized I was doing real spiritual harm to another soul.

Through all this, I began to ask myself: "Could I sit and watch someone I cared for literally die by inches? Could I cope with the reality that there was little or nothing I could do? How would I feel if I knew I was trapped in this situation and I could not walk away, that I must stay and endure the torture?" I don't think I would have the courage; yet, he does. What special grace from God must he have received to suffer so for my sake?

Of all the sins of my life, I believe this to be the worst. It will take some time before I resolve my guilt. I rejoice that someone (probably with the Lord's considerable help) was finally able to show me that there is more to this world than myself and my illness.

I also realize that this person who cares for me is not alone. The roster of those involved in direct care is increasing every day. We stand to lose the best of these heroes if we do not care for them as much as they have cared for us.

Kurt

I'd like to tell you about a friend of mine. His name was Kurt. Kurt was married and had a teenage daughter. Kurt owned his own business and was moderately successful. Several years ago, Kurt was in an automobile accident and lost his right leg from the knee down. But, with a prosthesis, he was able to remain active.

It was slightly over a year ago when Kurt also learned that he was positive for the AIDS virus. He contacted a local AIDS service organization and was enrolled in a support group called "Positive Images." I met Kurt in the support group and we became friends.

Kurt was very much impressed with the goal of the support group, which was to generate and maintain a positive mental attitude in the members.

As time progressed, the members of the group began to see some of their number become sick. Hospitalizations began to occur with alarming frequency. And then, one of the members died. A collection was taken for a memorial; then the group, with the encouragement of the group leaders, moved on to discussions of nutrition, sleep habits, and meditation. The group was collectively experiencing denial.

One member was not so inclined to sweep the death of a friend under a carpet of positive images. He was angry. Angry that someone had died. Angry that the group would not discuss death, sickness and debilitation, all fearful monoliths looming somewhere in the dark. Some of the meetings were disrupted with shouting, argument, and angry words.

And then Kurt got sick. Pneumonia. He was hospitalized and suffered a collapsed lung. He began to lose weight at an alarming rate. As he grew worse, his heart stopped and he was resuscitated. And then the virus began to affect his brain and he would complain of forgetting some event or conversation that had occurred just minutes before. Kurt came very close to death. But, eventually, he began to improve.

Toward the end of his recovery, I was also hospitalized. We found ourselves at opposite ends of the same hospital floor. We would sit for hours and talk and drink tea. The nurses desperately tried to track the whereabouts of their patients, but quickly learned that, when one of us was missing, he was with the other.

I will never forget that Kurt told me in the hospital that he knew he was going to "beat this thing." He was also angry with me for my behavior in our group meetings. I had been the angry one. He told me that "they (the group members) didn't need to hear about those things." By "things" he meant sickness and death.

After Kurt's brush with death, his attempts to "beat it" began to crumble as he began to realize that he had AIDS and that there was little likelihood that he was going to conquer the disease. He began to experience a severe depression. The doctors prescribed pills. His depression grew worse.

In our last telephone conversation, Kurt asked me why I thought the group wouldn't allow us to talk about the really scary things, like death. He told me that he thought they should.

Kurt was found one day, in his bed at home, dead. The cause of death was not listed in his obituary.

AIDS: A Manageable Disease?

I serve on the board of directors of a local organization which provides low-cost and subsidized housing to persons with AIDS. At a recent meeting, it became apparent that a new and dangerous trend is occurring in the world of AIDS. One of our board members characterized AIDS as being no longer an acute disease; it was, this person suggested, a disease that was quickly becoming chronic and manageable.

Anyone who has worked in this area for long, whether as a paid professional or as a volunteer, knows that it has been a long uphill struggle to get the government and the public to acknowledge, first the seriousness of the epidemic and, then, the need of those affected. Where we have met resistance from state, local, and federal agencies, we have met an even stonier silence from church groups and religious organizations. The difficulty with AIDS is that it raises not only the issues surrounding death and dying, but also issues like sexuality and substance abuse. These are all issues that make the American public very uncomfortable and often hostile.

And now, even those who have worked for long months in AIDS service organizations are characterizing the disease as non-acute, chronic, and manageable. For those who are uncomfortable with the issues, this is a perfect opportunity to shove AIDS a little further under the rug. It is, after all, only chronic — manageable. Why do we need to expend any special effort?

The reality is a little more grim.

Some weeks ago, I developed a sore throat and was having pain and difficulty swallowing. They found a massive infection of Candida (a yeast) that extended through the esophagus and even into the bowel. The treatment: a six-hour daily infusion of a drug that could, and did, cause severe tremors and chills. At one point, the intravenous needle went astray, and, before the infusion was stopped, my arm had been pumped to twice its normal size with a toxic drug. My arm was useless for about two weeks, and the pain was intense.

The AIDS virus has caused nerve damage in my legs, reducing my mobility. No one can tell me whether it will get worse.

I cannot take AZT because of anemia and a low white cell count. And, because of the nerve damage, I have been told that I cannot take the new drug DDI. Denied any drug that actually fights the virus, I could almost hear another nail being driven into my coffin.

I have been forced to wear adult diapers at night, and have bouts of diarrhea that no one can explain. My dignity has suffered a major jolt.

At one point, I cried that I was weary of always feeling bad and that maybe it would be better if it were all over. And then a friend told me the story of an elderly woman in his home town who had suffered a great deal before her death. When she was asked, "Do you need anything?" She would respond, "Just a little more Jesus."

So, at the board meeting, as I struggled to my feet and reached for my cane, I could only pray for "a little more Jesus" and mutter that the disease seemed pretty "acute" to me.

While we may have made progress in the treatment of the disease, we still have no cure. It is important, I think, to remember what the daily life of a person with AIDS is like and to refrain from giving some factions of our society any excuse for turning away. We are still struggling for services and research funds. We are still fighting prejudice and bigotry. People are still dying. From my vantage point, the disease seems very acute. AIDS will be truly manageable only when we have a cure.

"I'm Sorry You're Dying"

I recently experienced something quite unusual. At a meeting for an AIDS service organization, a woman with whom I had never before spoken, said to me, "I'm sorry that you are dying."

My immediate response was, "So am I!" I was taken by surprise, even a little shocked by her statement. But the more I consider the statement, the more I can appreciate it. It is direct, honest, and identifies the central issue of having AIDS. We *are* dying, and we need to acknowledge and accommodate that central truth. Once acknowledged, once accommodated, it does not suddenly disappear. This process is continuous.

This woman's statement to me was especially, and strangely, timely. I had been recently hospitalized and I came home very weak. I continue to lose weight despite lemon cake, lobster and melted butter, and boxes of chocolates. My legs have become unreliable and I am now forced to use a cane. It occurred to me that persons with AIDS no longer seem to die precipitously. With the advances in treating opportunistic infections like pneumocystis pneumonia, we don't die suddenly; we die slowly. It seems as if we grow gradually weaker, unable to metabolize any food, until we decide that we have suffered enough, and then we close our eyes and die. I have seen it too many time in the last year. The when is up to us — it comes at a time when we simply do not have any more energy to resist and we grow very tired.

I can honestly say that I have experienced very little depression, until recently. I suddenly just became tired of always feeling bad. I had been receiving a drug intravenously that caused shakes and chills. My arms had been punctured countless times. One arm had swollen to twice its size when one of the needles went astray. I had a transfusion for which they could find no needle site in either arm, so they had to go in near the shoulder. Within several days of coming home from the hospital, I awoke one morning and discovered that the entire right side of my face had swollen (another infection). So I had to begin taking antibiotics. The particular antibiotic prescribed causes diarrhea, on top of everything else. One night during this whole episode, I broke down. I cried in great, gut-wrenching sobs for an hour. I felt better afterwards. I was lucky; I had someone to hold me.

I am writing about these experiences because I firmly believe that the quality of my life since the diagnosis has been greatly enhanced by an honest, direct realization that I do have a terminal illness, that I have maybe a year (by the doctor's latest estimate), and that I will die. I have little tolerance for those who don't want to talk about death — I think they are really cheating themselves. We can become bores; we think about AIDS all of the time. We want to talk about it. But my death from AIDS does not seem to be a particularly popular topic of conversation at cocktail parties.

I suppose that this chapter is an appeal. Death from AIDS is hard enough. If you have a friend or a loved one with AIDS, do them a great service and help them to talk about the hard subjects. Let them feel that they can talk about their fears. Hold them when they need to cry. Be with them through the terror, the depression, the tears.

And, pray for us all.

Baking Bread for the Soul

My faith and my prayer life have always been fairly generic. They included the basics, but there weren't any fireworks or great flashes of religious fervor. I believed in God and the Sacraments, and understood the major lessons of the Gospels. Prayer was mostly for Sunday and whenever I found myself in serious trouble. But, for the most part, I was a very practical person, and I have always done better with a cookbook than a prayer book. You mix these ingredients this way and you get that. Prayer books were just too indefinite for my taste.

Then came the diagnosis of AIDS. I knew there were going to be some changes in the way I experienced my faith: "There are no atheists in foxholes." But I was not prepared for the actuality. The outpouring of grace that I have experienced has changed everything, from the smallest item to the really big things like my perception of who and what God is. There is now little resemblance between what I thought my faith was and what it has become.

Shortly after the diagnosis, I remember going to the chapel at the hospital. When I knelt before the altar, I could not find any words. So all I did was cry. It was a valuable lesson, and I've found that meaningful prayer, for me, consists mainly of silence. In order to hear God, I had to shut up first. I know this may sound a bit odd, but when I approach the Lord in silence, I feel a sense of warmth and comfort. I suppose it could be described as a "presence."

Before these changes in my spiritual life, my personality was basically cold and aloof. I firmly believe that the grace that I have received has turned my soul outward. I now find myself talking with strangers in line at the grocery or at the post office. And now I find myself much more interested in others and their lives than I am in my own problems. My pastor, after a recent visit, left saying that he felt as if he had been ministered to instead of the other way around. I feel very good about that.

This turning outward seems to have the effect of attracting others to me. I am surrounded by those who really care. And if I ever had the desire to see Christ in the flesh, I have to look no further than the hands that are extended to me daily.

I know that I have done absolutely nothing to deserve this — which makes it all the more wondrous. Any formal prayers that I may say now are likely to be prayers of praise and thanksgiving.

So in terms of cookbook religion, take one part of prayerful silence, two parts of trust, a sprinkle of tears, and mix gently. You don't really have to do anything else, because the Lord will take care of the rising, the kneading, and the baking.

Earthly Attachments

Toward the beginning of my journey with AIDS, I spent considerable time thinking about death in general. When I felt fairly comfortable, I spent some time thinking about my own death in particular. I thought that I had reached a rather uneasy peace with death. I realized that I had developed certain earthly attachments that I would simply have to give up. I would not become a vice-president at the bank. I probably would not win the lottery and become a world traveler. Anyway, doesn't my religion teach that I should not become too enamored of impermanent, imperfect things in this life?

And then AIDS wrought it's indelible changes on my life. AIDS did not just change my life, it transformed my life. From an early age I have wanted to write. My first faltering attempts at age twenty were not met with great applause. Now, I am writing daily — and people are actually reading what I write. I have always had a difficult (sometimes hostile) relationship with my mother. Now she calls weekly, and I am able to tell her that I love her. Some of the most brilliant and compassionate people in the world are those who are involved with AIDS and other social issues. Now I can count some of them as my friends. And being officially disabled, and not required to be on the job Monday through Friday,

I have the time to dedicate myself to work that is truly important. I am no longer just a volunteer.

I was hospitalized recently. When I was released, I realized that this episode had done some permanent damage. Some vital piece of me had been taken away, and I could feel its loss. In a follow-up visit with my doctor, he told me quite honestly that I was not doing as well as he would have liked. He said that he was worried about me. He also asked if I was scared. It took me fully two days to realize that, yes, I am scared. I am very scared. I also realize that I have replaced an old set of "earthly attachments" with a new set. I realize that I will eventually lose the ability to do the work that I love so much, that I will have to say good-bye to my new, wonderful friends. And, once again, I find myself mourning. It is an overwhelming melancholy, a deep sadness. I have never known anyone with AIDS who has not required some time to mourn for themselves.

One of my all-time favorite songs is sung by Emmylou Harris. It has the unmistakable flavor of the Ozark mountains and all of the rich religious tradition of that region. The title is "When He Calls." The refrain goes something like this: "When He calls, I'm gonna live with Jesus. In His Kingdom He welcomes everyone. I shall fear no more earthly perils, He will carry me home."

It is difficult for me to listen to this song now. And when I do, the tears begin to flow. I have been caught several times by friends who are lovingly concerned, but mystified by my behavior. They want to know, "What's wrong?" How can I explain that I am mourning? How can I tell them that I will miss them and all of the beautiful things in this life? How can I tell them how much I will miss coffee at sunrise and hymns on Sunday and lilacs in the spring? How can I tell them how much I will miss their smile and touch?

How do I tell them that I do not want to say good-bye?

Father

Having AIDS is a lot of work. You find yourself no longer able to ignore or put off things that you have avoided for years. Somehow, a terminal illness forces you to resolve those relationships and hurts from years past that have hung around in the background like cobwebs. You don't really want to, because it can be very painful, but you feel an unrelenting urge to clear away those cobwebs. I realized some time ago that it does no good to resist the urge. You might as well get it over with.

So, there is the problem of my father. My parents were divorced when I was about fourteen. I had not known at the time that my father apparently had a penchant for ladies other than my mother, and that he was not particularly skilled in hiding his various rendezvous. As you can imagine, the relationship between by father and mother was quite stormy. My father was also a dreamer and had incurred some substantial debts. His solution to his debt problem was to move. So for most of my junior and high school years, we moved from city to city. This didn't encourage emotional stability in me or in my brothers and sister. It seemed as if there was always a new school, a new playground bully. I put on weight and became a "fat kid," and withdrew.

After the divorce, my father just disappeared. My mother and my grandparents tried in vain to track him down for child support. But often the only address was a post office box. So my mother was forced to raise four children on about eighty dollars a week. It was hard, and my brothers and sister and I didn't hear a great deal of positive talk about my father.

My relationship with my father was a disappointment to both of us. He felt that I should play football, go deer hunting, and so forth. I had no aptitude for sports, especially with my weight problem. And hunting and fishing literally turned my stomach — so badly that there was no way I could hide it from him. By the time I was a freshman in high school, I knew that I was a large disappointment to him, and that I was just not the son whom he had wanted.

Later, after his disappearance, I began to develop my anger. I had no money for new school clothes; I had no money to go out for hamburgers with friends. And it was all my father's fault, especially if you listened to my mother.

So I come to this point in my life, not really knowing my father, feeling a deep anger and mistrust. But the really painful part is that somewhere down deep, I know I love him; I always have, despite the hurt. And now I have to tell this man, whom I don't really know, that I love him. I don't mind admitting that I'm scared to death and that this will be one of the hardest things I've every done.

I've been encouraged. My sister told him that I had AIDS and he has called twice since. So, maybe there's hope. If ever I needed to rely on my God for strength and courage, this is it. But I have a hunch that this is just the sort of thing that the Holy Spirit does really well. Love conquers all? When it comes to my father, I'm not so sure. But I'm willing to give it a shot. Pray for me.

My Eulogy

This is a temptation that I could not resist — having the very last word. Besides, I'm leaving no great legacy. I haven't left millions to charity or an art collection to a museum. So there are a few things I would like to tell you that I think are very important. Let them be my legacy.

You all know that my death was the result of AIDS. Some of you have heard about AIDS and my particular troubles for several years. I suppose that I became something of a bore over that time. But your willingness to listen to my constant banter about AIDS has helped me greatly in coming to terms with what has now happened, my death.

At the doorway of death, I find myself very poor. I have only my faith in God and the love that many of you have given me. I have no particular claim to a righteous life or good works of any note. I do have some baggage; we call them sins. Aside from that, I approach death with very little.

I have no idea what this new adventure of death will be like. My faith tells me that it is not the end. I really have no idea whether I will see a blinding light, whether there is such a place as heaven, or whether I might actually qualify for a pair of wings (or the reverse). It will be a true adventure. I want you all to know, however, that whatever death may bring, I will always love you and will think of you often. If it is possible, as I believe it is, I will pray for you and keep you in my heart always. I look forward to seeing you again when you begin your great adventure.

The most difficult thing for me in writing this eulogy is the picture of the grief that some of you will be suffering. It is very hard for me to bear the thought of the sadness in my mother's face, in Richard's eyes. I can't bear the thought of being responsible for such sadness. But, as with the disease that finally claimed me, there isn't much that I can do to help.

Death from AIDS is a long, slow process. Painful, soul-wrenching, debilitating. So be glad for me in this small thing: my suffering has ended and I have gone on to better things. I hope that you, having been with me during this time, will remember and offer your care and love to others who are suffering.

The greatest part of my legacy is a thing which a special friend described to me as "The Embracing of Souls." It is something that many of us only experience once or twice during our lifetime. It describes those very special people who come into our lives at odd, unpredictable times. Love flows between two spirits like water in a stream. It is a very special gift from God. In fact, I believe that this "embracing of souls" is the Spirit of God working in our lives. St. John must have known about the "embracing of souls" when he said that "God is Love." And I have been blessed enough to experience it. I have no idea why I have been so blessed; I can only accept with gratitude.

I have to say something about two of the very special people in my life: my mother and Richard. My mother raised four children on her own with no money and very little support from anyone else. And she did this during a time when issues like child-care, child support, divorce and working mothers were treated like dirty little secrets to be hidden away. She took us through adolescence with absolutely no cooperation from us. I remember times when she had to scrape the bottom of her purse for pennies so we could have bread and milk for dinner. Of course, those were the days when a loaf of bread was twenty cents. It is hard for me now to imagine the anguish and fear that she must have experienced. But she did it, and I love her for it. She has lost her parents, her husband, and now a son. It seems so awful to me that someone who has done so much should have to suffer so. I love you, mom.

And then there is Richard, bull-headed, impossible, a mother-hen, but one of the few people I have ever known who has absolutely no malice in his heart. Richard is one of those people who simply doesn't understand hatred or cruelty or lies or deceit of any sort. He really just doesn't understand it. Thank God he doesn't. Imagine the special grace that it must take to suffer as he has. He has been forced to watch me waste away unto death, and there was absolutely nothing he could do to change the course of the disease, absolutely nothing. He has given me injections when I have been shaking so badly that I couldn't inject myself. He has sat with me for hours in the emergency room after working a full midnight shift. He has supported me, cared for me, and loved me while he watched me die. The bond between us (our "embracing of souls") is strong. Death cannot break it. And if there is such a thing as earning a place in heaven, he has earned his place many times over.

My suffering has ended. But I want you all to know that the best you can do in this life is to experience an embracing of souls. In that, you experience God himself. It will prepare you for whatever suffering you may have to experience. It will allow you to bear up, and even to give thanks in the midst of the suffering.

Until I see you again, all my love.

Endnotes

[1] John E. Fortunato, *AIDS, The Spiritual Dilemma*, (Harper & Row, San Francisco (c) 1987), page 84.

[2] *Ibid.*, page 69.

[3] *Ibid.*, page 18.

[4] *Ibid.*, pages 85-86.

[5] Louis Evely, translated by Edmond Bonin, *That Man Is You*, (Paulist Press, New York, (c) 1964), page 20.

For More Information

If you are a person with AIDS, have a loved one with AIDS, or are called to minister to persons with AIDS, you may find the following organizations helpful in your search for information and support.

National AIDS Information Clearinghouse, 1-800-458-5231. This national organization offers free publications and listings of AIDS-related community groups throughout the United States.

National Council of Churches, NCC AIDS Task Force, 475 Riverside Dr., Room 572, New York, NY 10115. An AIDS resource packet for congregations can be ordered for a $5.00 processing fee.

United Methodist Board of Discipleship, Discipleship Resources, P.O. Box 189, Nashville, TN 37202. A study guide, *AIDS and the Ministry of the Church*, is available from this denominational organization.

United Methodist Board of Global Ministries, 475 Riverside Dr., Room 350, New York, NY 10115. This group offers a variety of resources to churches or conferences interested in AIDS ministries.

About the Author

Terry Boyd, the father of one teenage son, was raised in Nebraska, Idaho. A Micro-Computer specialist working with a small savings and loan association, Terry was formerly a Navy medic with part of his service years spent in Viet Nam.

Since his diagnosis of AIDS, Terry has been active in the effort to help others with AIDS and has worked closely with national and local AIDS groups. A member of the United Methodist Missouri-East Conference AIDS Task Force, Terry is also a volunteer for St. Louis Effort for AIDS, a local AIDS service organization.

Terry, who had never received much religious training as a child, began his spiritual journey at the age of twenty, when he became a Roman Catholic. He spent a year in a Benedictine monastery, but eventually became disillusioned and left the church. Years later, a friend invited Terry to attend Lafayette Park United Methodist Church in St. Louis, where he is now a member. It was to that church's pastor that he first revealed his diagnosis of AIDS. To his relief, the congregation's reaction has been overwhelmingly supportive, strengthening Terry's faith and lightening his pain and depression.

"I truly feel that, even in the face of AIDS, I have been blessed tremendously," Terry writes.

www.ingramcontent.com/pod-product-compliance
Lightning Source LLC
Chambersburg PA
CBHW060854050426
42453CB00008B/974